Surviving

the Storm

Ti'Ocea Hagins

Dedication

This book is dedicated to me...

because I faced the storm and survived.

Acknowledgements

I dedicate this book to the ones I love the most. My Family! Mom, dad, sister, brothers, my son and my fiancé. You guys have struggled through some tough times with me and without you guys, I don't know where I would be.

To my Mother (LaTanya): Sometimes things may seem rough for a season. But just know through this journey we call life, no matter what happens, I love you more than life itself and I could not have asked for a better mother. We will make it through anything.

To my Dad (Cameron): I love you more than all the stars in the sky. I thank you for being there to support me and taking care of me even if you didn't agree with everything I did. People may not understand, but you truly are a Father anyone would be lucky to have.

To my Sister and Brothers (Chasity, Tyler and Cameron): I love you all to the moon and back again. Thanks for being my rock when I truly needed you all and never asking any questions. I could not have asked for better siblings.

To my Friends and the rest of my family who supported me through my good and tough times: Just know I love you all with my heart and I thank you for being there to support me and being by myside every step of the way.

And last but certainly not least...

To my son & fiancé - (Darien & Jhace). I love you both to the moon and back again. Thanks for giving me the strength to fight so hard for something to come back to. I was ready to give up at one point and let go, but God kept me here on his earth just for you. I love you both with all my heart and soul and always remember it's US AGAINST THE WORLD!!!!!

I love you all!

Table of Contents

Introduction

I remember when I first started to get sick. It was a rainy day out in Canandaigua, New York. Working for Finger Lakes Developmental Disabilities Service Office in the State of New York can be very challenging and physically and emotionally draining. Especially because we work with individuals with developmental disabilities. I was at work doing the second half of my double shift, when I started to feel sick. My throat began to hurt, my ears began to throb, and my throat started to become dry. My boss was out taking the clients shopping, so I could not do anything until she returned home. I was going to ask if I could go home and lay down to see if I could fight this thing off before it got any worse. I wasn't going to make it through the day and needed to leave there and fast.

Just as I was about to call her on the phone to ask her if I can leave for the day, she came walking through the door with the clients and bags in her hand. It must have shown on my face that I was not feeling good, because before I could even speak anything, she spoke up.

"Ti'Ocea are you ok? You do not look so good."

"No Ash. I am not feeling well. My throat hurts, my ears are throbbing, and my eyes are starting to become pink. Do you mind if I take the day off and go home and rest?" I asked her, trying to do it the right way because she can be a little nasty and I was going to leave, even if she had said no.

"Sure, go ahead," she said with an attitude. I knew from her tone and prior instances that she did not care too much for black people, but I wasn't feeling well enough to deal with her ba-foolery that day.

"Call me tomorrow if you are still not feeling well and I will use the time you have for your days out," she said to me as I was gathering my things to head home.

I went to the back office to gather my things, finish my notes, and sign out to head home. I was hoping and praying that I could make it home in peace, since I was all the way out in Canandaigua, NY and had to drive all the way back to the city of Rochester. "Thanks, Ash!" I said to her as I continued to say thank you and my goodbyes to all my co-workers. They had allowed me to rest myself that day and picked up my portion of the work. I was truly grateful, because I was no good. Little did I know that would be my last time seeing them and my "see you tomorrow's" would be no more.

Someone help me! Someone help me please! I am being taken. Mommy... Daddy help!

Those are the thoughts that were going through my head as I was rolling on something that seemed like a cart going somewhere unfamiliar. My eyes began to flutter, and I began to see things quickly. I must have been medicated, but just not enough because I was beginning to awaken. Something was wrong, and I was determined to figure it out. I tried to move my arms and legs and realized I was being held down. Help me, someone help! I tried to scream, but something was stuck in my throat and I couldn't scream for help.

Now I am worried. Someone had me and I needed to get out of here fast. I started to move my legs and arms to break free from my grip, but the restraints were too tight and too strong. Someone help me? I tried screaming again and opened my eyes to see where I was, but just as I was trying to get them fully open, I was hit with this thing called sleep and my fight to get free had just killed me.

I came into the hospital to be treated for the flu and ended up with machines working to keep me alive. I had been to the doctor's office a thousand times and nothing seemed to be working. My nose had an infection; my ears had an infection, and I had pink eye in both eyes.

Family and friends were gathering in the conference room at the hospital. Some were sick to their stomachs, others felt like they couldn't breathe. No one was eating or drinking anything. You could hear prayers to GOD being spoken throughout the room. Surgeons and Doctors were coming into the room to make sure that everyone was ok. They brought sandwich trays and drinks to the room so that someone would eat something, but no one could touch anything.

"Mr. and Mrs. Johnson," Doctor Jackson spoke as he walked into the waiting room full of worried faces.

"Ye-es," my mom said faintly as she waited for the doctor to speak.

"I need to be completely honest with you. It does not look good." With no response, he continued. "Her colon is perforated, and she needs an emergency surgery immediately. Whether, I perform the surgery or not, your daughter has a twenty percent chance of surviving."

All you could hear in the room was gasping. No one could breathe, let alone say anything. Dad was in the corner throwing up uncontrollably and mommy felt her whole world had collapsed as she had to grip on to her chair, because her legs were weakening beneath her.

"Should I proceed?" Dr. Jackson asked, but no one was able to answer him as everyone was too busy praying trying to make sure that I stayed alive.

"Shall I proceed?" Dr. Jackson asked again, needing to get to the surgery room as soon as possible to try and save my life.

All Mom and Dad could do was nod their head yes. They were so sick that the hospital was going to admit them to the emergency room. Doctor

Jackson started walking towards the door and looked back towards the family.

"Mr. and Mrs. Johnson, I promise I will do everything I can to save your daughter's life," he said without waiting for a response. With that, he walked out of the room ready to prepare for a surgery that may or may not save a young woman's life.

Come with me as I take you on the journey of my survival one day at a time!

Chapter 1

Deep in a Ditch

My name is Ti'Ocea and I am 29 years old from Rochester, New York. Rochester, is a city on the southern shore of Lake Ontario in Western N.Y. I come from a city where drugs and violence has taken many lives. Rochester is home to many; families of celebrities, athletes, concerned citizens and parents. But the streets belong to those that have taken over from drugs and murder. Compared to other cities, Rochester is ranked number 16 in its homicide rates.

I'm what many would call a "good girl." I've never been hooked on, let alone taken any drugs. I went to a catholic high school and the only problems I have ever had with the law are traffic violations. Being raised in a two-parent household has shaped me into dealing with the different encounters that I have faced in my life. I cannot complain and say that I had to live a rough or tough lifestyle. In actuality, I grew up living what most would say was a "good life." I lived in nice homes, received the best education and played in every sport that I didn't quit in one day. My parents made sure that their children grew up not wanting for anything. No, we were not rich by far, but they made sure that we didn't have to struggle or live a horrific lifestyle. So, they did everything they could to make sure we were happy and had whatever we needed.

—

I was a normal person, living a normal life. But what is normal? How can anyone define normal in this world today? Well you can't. Normal means different things for different people. My normal and your normal are not the same and will never be the same. Maybe this all began when I was hit by an 18-wheeler and my life changed.

I was on my way to work one day driving in West Henrietta, NY in my 2001 Volvo S40. Now everyone who lives in Rochester knows that West Henrietta has three lanes both ways due to the heavy amount of traffic that it receives daily. An 18-wheeler in the far left-hand lane, started to make a wide right turn across the lanes into a store. I slammed on my brakes and laid on my horn. Nothing seemed to work, because before I knew it "boom," the front of the truck hit me on my driver side door, and my car flew up and slammed into a ditch.

I felt my life flash before my eyes. I really couldn't believe what just happened. I had blood on my face and glass shattered all over me. My legs were crunched up to the steering wheel and I couldn't move my arms. Glass stuck out of my leg and I felt myself gasping for air. The car was smoking, and I was panicking trying to get out, thinking *"this car is about to catch on fire."*

"Ma'am are you ok?" I heard a woman say but couldn't see her face.

"No, I am scared and in pain. Can you please call my mom?" I asked, as I couldn't move my arm because it was broken from the impact. The lady called my mother and normally she never answers unknown numbers, but for some reason she had a feeling that this call needed to be answered. Her feeling was right!

"Hello!" my mother answered on the other end of the line, confused as to who was calling her phone and what they wanted.

"Hello ma'am, my name is Carol and I am with your daughter. She was hit by an 18-wheeler and asked me to call you."

"OMG, Cam!" I heard my mother scream on the other end of Carol's phone, while hearing the sirens in the background. I was thanking God that the ambulance was on its way.

"Cam, we have to go now! Thank you for your call ma'am. Please stay with my daughter until I arrive," my mother asked the lady as they were nearing the end of the call.

Out the corner of my eye, I saw a fireman standing at my window. *Fire policemen is what I used to call them.* I couldn't move my neck because it was stuck from the impact of the crash.

"Ma'am, this is the fire department. Are you ok?" I heard him ask but couldn't see his face.

"No sir, I am in a lot of pain and I can't feel my legs. Please get me out of here!" I pleaded to him.

"Ma'am, you will be fine. We are getting ready to get you out. I am putting this jacket over your head, so that we can cut your door and the roof to get you out. Please be still, we will be quick," he said to me as I heard a machine biting into my door. I guess that's what they call the jaws of life. They had to use it to get me out because I was so far deep inside the ditch that it took six men to get me out of that car and on to the stretcher.

"Baby are you ok?" I heard my mother and father ask as the paramedics put me on the stretcher taking me to the ambulance.

"No, I am in so much pain," I said to them.

"We will meet you at the hospital," they said to me as I was being loaded into the ambulance and on my way.

I was so distraught and in pain that I never got the time to thank the lady who had took her time out to wait with me until I made it into the ambulance. She was truly a blessing. At the hospital, they started running test after test, blood work after blood work and doping me up on medicine so I wouldn't be in so much pain and could rest with ease. I had to receive stitches in my head where the glass from the impact cut me deep. I thought to myself, *"now I have to live with scars forever"*. Not that having scars was a problem, it was just dis-heartening that I had bruises and scars all over my body. My legs were all scratched up and my arms had some as well. What's weird is that the right leg that has a tattoo of prayer hands and my grandmother's name never got a single scratch. I guess that was a sign that I was covered by the blood of Jesus.

Romans 8:28 (NKJV)

"And we know that all things work together for good to those who love God, to those who are the called according to His purpose."

Chapter 2

You Should be Dead

It took six long months to recover from that accident. I had to go through many months and hours of physical therapy, all while wearing a cast on my leg and arm that had become sprained and broken in the accident. I was always going back and forth to doctors appointments and given orders for bed rest so that I could heal faster.

After getting the ok from my doctor to return to work and school, I ended up going back to work the next day for the State of New York (FLDDSO) and going back to finishing my classes at Monroe Community College. I was studying Criminal Justice in school and really enjoyed the major I had chosen. It was something that I always wanted to do since I was a little girl. I enjoyed every bit of it, and I was determined to graduate no matter the obstacles that came my way, I was not going to let anything stop me from accomplishing my dreams and achieving my goals. I excelled in school and exceeded expectations at work. I was enjoying getting back to normalcy, until life happened and turned my dreams into nightmares and my life into hell. Well... what felt like hell.

—

It was Easter Sunday 2012, and all the family had come over to enjoy an Easter dinner and relax together. We made baked mac and cheese, cabbage, rice and gravy, chitterlings, dressing, gumbo, cornbread, candy yams, ham, and sweet potato pie. Now normally we don't cook like this on Easter, but the family decided that it was time to have a family get together and just enjoy one another. The approaching holiday was as good a time as any for us to enjoy spending the day together.

The food had just been set on the table and everyone had been called to come wash their hands so we can eat. Children filed to the bathroom, while the adults lined up at the sink, but for some reason I never moved from the couch. I slowly got up and made my way to the sink to wash my hands and just didn't feel good. Something was not right, but I couldn't figure out what was going on with me. I made my plate and sat at the table with my family as they started to say grace and bless the food.

"Amen," everyone said, as forks and spoons started being lifted to dig in. For some reason I just couldn't eat. As a matter of fact, I couldn't even pick up my fork and I didn't know why. Then I felt it. My hands went numb and I couldn't feel a thing. My mom knew something was wrong because I always eat and this time I just couldn't.

"Baby, what's wrong, why are you not eating?" I heard my mother ask from across the table. The only thing I could say was, "I can't feel my hands. I don't feel good."

Well, I guess you know after those words they made a call to my doctor to figure out what was wrong. My doctor was awesome. She was always someone who cared about her patients and did everything she could to make sure that her patients got the best care any time of the day and week. She was my family's doctor, starting with my grandmother, then my parents, and finally me. Dr. Heather Lenior specialized in treating an extensive variety of disorders and illnesses that affect adults. She received her medical degree from the University of Rochester and has been practicing medicine for more than twenty years.

I was Dr. Heather Lenior's second to last patient of the day. She had just finished up with another patient, when I heard a knock at the door and the door swung open.

"Hello, Dr. Heather Lenior, how are you?" I stated to her as she came in with her computer and took a seat in her chair next to me. She was very thorough, so she took a lot of notes and made sure that she dotted all her I's and crossed all her T's.

"Ti'Ocea what is going on with you? You don't look so well," she stated to me as she looked between her computer and myself.

"Dr. Heather Lenior, I do not know what is going on," I stated as my mother explained to her what happened on Easter Sunday.

She started typing something in her computer, as I sat there waiting for her to come up with a solution to find some results as to what was going on.

"Let's check you out to see what's going on," she stated as she started to do her exam on my body. "Does this hurt?" she asked as she examined me.

"Yes, that hurts right there," I responded to her as she motioned for me to lay back on the table again.

She finished her exam and started typing some notes in her computer, as we sat there waiting for her to come up with a solution. "I think I want you to go see neurology, just to check on your hand and figure out why you cannot move it. I am going to also send over a prescription to help with the pain to see if we can't get you to feeling better, until we know exactly what is going on. I want to see you back in my office in a week, so make sure you let the front desk know so we can get that scheduled for you."

"Ok. Sounds good," I replied as I got down from the exam table and started to head out into the hallway toward check out. After leaving the doctor's office, I had my appointment with neurology scheduled two days later and my follow up appointment one week later. I was told to just take it easy, take my meds and get all the rest possible. Somehow, that last part was hard to do.

I went to the neurology appointment referred by my PCP, who in the interim, determined that I had carpel tunnel and had explained to me that I needed to wear a brace for a few weeks to see if we could correct the problem. Little did he know this was just the beginning. As the days and weeks passed, I became sicker and sicker. I was losing weight constantly. I was in excruciating pain and because of it, I could barely sleep. Something was wrong, but not one doctor could figure out what it was.

I went from doctor to doctor, hospital to hospital, specialist to specialist and every hour and day that passed, I was getting worse and worse. Every test that was taken, kept coming back normal. No one could figure out why I was getting sicker with normal test results and it was something that we were fighting daily to figure out. Doctors ended up putting me on a steroid because I was dropping weight left and right, but that ended up being a failure, because I just continued to lose weight instead of gaining.

Everyone that I had seen just felt as if they were ready to give up and had exhausted every option they could, but my parents would not take no for an answer. They wanted results and so did I, but I was in too much pain and too sick to fight as they were. Someone was going to tell them what was wrong with their child. It was a nightmare trying to figure out why I was getting so sick and why the medicine that was being prescribed was not making any positive results. In fact, the medication was hurting more than helping.

Every night and day that I laid my head down, I just felt as if I wanted to die. I was in so much pain and no one could tell us why. What was wrong with me? And why am I getting sicker and sicker? It was a question that so many of us wanted answered, but no one could give us anything until one person decided to do something new to see if they could get some results.

I went back to see Dr. Heather Lenior since I was getting worse since the neurology appointment. As I was sitting there in thought waiting in the room to be seen, there was a knock at the door.

"Ti'Ocea how are doing today?" Dr. Lenior asked as she took a seat in her chair with her computer ready to get to work. She saw how I was deteriorating right in front of her eyes.

"No one seems to know what is going on with me. I have taken test after test and been to doctor after doctor. I just don't know what else to do," I stated weakly. She continued typing some notes, as I sat there patiently waiting for her to come up with a solution. She was my last hope since no one else seemed to know how to properly diagnosis the issue.

"I think I want you to schedule an MRI and see if this will show us what is going on with you. We seem to have exhausted every other option possible," Dr. Lenior stated to me as she continued to speak. "I also want to prescribe you some different medication to see if we can control the pain a little better, until we figure out what the cause of this sickness is. I also would like to see you back in my office in one week after the scan, just to come up with a plan to make sure that we get you back to your normal health and self again," Dr. Heather Lenior stated as she typed a few more notes and asked me to get on the table so that she could examine me.

"Ok, Ti'Ocea, let's get this MRI scheduled with the imaging center and then we will work on a plan from there. I also would like to see you back here in a week, just to keep a close eye on you." Dr. Heather Lenior stated as she handed me my patient care plan.

"Sounds good," I replied as I got down from the exam table and started to head out into the hall-way toward check out.

It was crazy because out of all the doctors and hospitals I had visited over the last several weeks, no one ever thought to do an MRI to see if they can find out what was wrong. I had scheduled CT scans, but nothing was found on them. I probably could have been better if someone scheduled an MRI in the first place. We didn't know if this was going to work, but the only thing we had left to lean on was our faith.

For those who have trouble with medical terminology and have no clue what an MRI (Medical resonance imaging) is, it's a medical imaging technique that is used in radiology to form pictures of the anatomy and the physiological process of the body in both health and disease.

I walked through the doors of the imaging center nervous because I did not know whether we would leave with answers or if we would be back to square one and that scared me more than anything. Shortly after check-in, I was called up to start my prep before they brought me into my MRI scan. My stomach had started to turn, not only from me being nervous, but also because I hated drinking that nasty stuff, like they couldn't do any better. I said a prayer to God to reveal some results to help us determine what was wrong. I drank the prep and even though it always made me nauseous, I held my breath and took the whole bottle. I was brought back out to the waiting room to wait with my mother until a room was available for me and my prep had kicked in.

About forty-five minutes later, I was taken back into the room to start my IV and get ready for the scan. It took about an hour. Once the scan was finished, my mother and I checked out and headed out of the door, hoping that we will get some results sooner than later. We walked through the parking lot to our car and started to pull off heading back home. Not even two minutes after we pulled off, I received a call from an unknown number. Now normally I do not answer unknown numbers but for some reason, this feeling I had, told me to answer it but what I didn't know is what was being said on the other line would change my life.

"Hello," I stated to the unknown person on the other end of my line.

"Hello, this is Dr. Santiago at the imaging center. May I please speak with Ms. Ti'Ocea Hagins?" the doctor asked. I was now getting concerned about this call. "Hello, Dr. Santiago. This is she. How may I help you?

"Ms. Hagins, I need you to go to the hospital immediately." Dr. Santiago stated as I now began to panic trying to figure out what was wrong with me and why I was being told to go to hospital.

"Dr. may I ask what is wrong? Why do I need to go to the hospital?" I asked as Mom already had begun driving in that direction.

"Ma'am just go to the hospital and you will be advised from there," Dr. Santiago stated as she disconnected the call.

Speeding through the streets of New York, Mom and I were bobbing in and out of traffic trying to get to the emergency department. Within ten minutes we arrived at the hospital. Going in, I felt lightheaded and sick, I ended up having to be pushed in a wheelchair because my legs became very weak and felt as if they were going to collapse on me. It might have just been the nerves, but I needed to be safe on this one, so being pushed was the best and safest option for me.

We walked into a packed emergency room. Luckily, Dr. Santiago had already called and updated them on my diagnosis because they quickly checked me in, took my vitals, asked simple questions and led me into a vacant room right away. As, we got settled into my room, thoughts were going in and out of my head as I wondered and pondered on every possible scenario of why I could be this sick, praying to get answers fast. Just as I was about to ask my mother a question, the doctor walked into the room, and our hearts dropped as we waited patiently to hear why I was asked to be rushed to the hospital.

"Ms. Hagins, I am Dr. Love a physician assistant here under Dr. John. I would ask how you are but looking at you I can see that you could be doing much better," she said to me as I just looked at her wanting the results not wanting to hear anything else she had to say at the moment. Dr. Love was looking through my chart as we sat there impatiently waiting for her to tell us why they had us there. Dr. Love looked up from the computer and into our direction.

"Dr. Santiago called and gave us a brief synopsis, but before I tell you what is going on, can you please tell me what has been going on with you?" Dr. Love asked looking between my mom and me. Before I could speak, my mom chimed in and explained to the doctor what was going on and what they thought was the problem in the beginning. Anytime I go to the doctor or appointments, my mom tends to do that, so I became used to it. My family has always been very passionate about our health and if anything, seemed out of place, they were the first ones to speak up and speak out. I wasn't complaining though; I was in no mood to talk I was in too much pain and felt way too weak to even speak to anyone.

After speaking with my mother, Dr. Love then wrote some notes and looked between the two of us and then back at me. The reason you were told to be rushed to the hospital is because the MRI found blood clots in your legs that have traveled to your lungs. In medical terminology they are called pulmonary embolisms and it looks as if there are a plethora of them that have clogged your lungs," Dr. Love said to us as she continued to speak.

"Ma'am, I don't know how you are waking up out of your sleep, but you are one lucky woman. With the number of pulmonary embolisms in your lungs, I don't see how you are falling asleep and waking up. You really should be dead." Dr. Love stated as she begun to type something into her computer. As she typed, tears began to fall down our faces, because we didn't need to think twice about how I was waking up from my sleep, we knew it was no one but God.

Ever since Dr. Love explained to us what the results were, there seemed to be so many mixed feelings. On one hand, we were ecstatic that we had finally got some answers as to why I was so sick, but on the other hand it was heart breaking to know that these pulmonary embolisms could have been the cause of my death and no one would have never known.

For those of you who do not know medical terminology such as myself, a pulmonary embolism is a blockage in one of the pulmonary arteries in your lungs. It is caused by a blood clot that has traveled to your lungs from the legs, or rarely, other parts of the body. This is caused deep vein thrombosis (DVT). The most common symptoms of pulmonary embolisms are shortness of breath, chest pain and cough. I had none of those symptoms. I was just walking around and getting sicker all while having clots clogging my lungs and arteries.

To think that I could have went to sleep and never woke up was scary, but I knew that I was covered by the blood of Jesus and he was by my side. When things like this happen, the only thing that you have to lean on is your faith in Jesus Christ.

Isaiah 54:17 (NKJV)

"No weapon formed against you shall prosper, And every tongue which rises against you in judgment You shall condemn…"

Chapter 3

From Pulmonary Embolisms to Auto Immune Disease

I hated the hospital. I hated staying overnight there even more. But it was something that Dr. Love had requested, so they could monitor me closely and start me on my treatment. Not only did they have me on Coumadin the blood thinner, they also had me on Heparin shots that had to be given in my stomach everyday two times a day. As if I wasn't in enough pain already, and now they wanted to give me shots in my stomach. Ughhh… That was the thought going through my head as I lay in the hospital getting poked and bruised every five minutes, or so it felt.

The overnight stay in the hospital felt like an eternity. I didn't get discharged until late afternoon. You would think that after they found the blood clots that I would be healed quickly, and things would have gotten better. Well they didn't! Things had gotten worse for me and it didn't take long. We thought that we had found the reason of why I was becoming so sick, but that had just been the beginning of the pain and worry.

For anyone who has never had a blood clot or never experienced it with a family member or close friend, then you have yet to begin to understand the affects and effects blood clots and the medications to treat them can have on your life. I was sent home with a prescription for Heparin shots (blood thinner) and Coumadin (warfarin) something that can potentially be very harmful to my body, especially if not used correctly. Heparin is an anticoagulant or blood thinner that's helps to prevent the formation of blood. Coumadin treats blood clots, but also lowers your chance of blood clots forming in your body. For those of you who have ever been on Coumadin or Heparin shots, then you know exactly where I am coming from. Coumadin can be very dangerous and life saving at the same time. Yes, it protects against blood clots from forming in your body, however, the risks of bleeding out if you accidently cut yourself or fall is extremely dangerous.

Imagine being told that you can never have children or if you fall you can potentially bleed out internally and may never know it while being on this medication. Scary ain't it? Now, I know that there are many young people and people in general going through similar situations, or even worse, there are those who did not live to tell their story. Yet, when you are going through something and God turns a deadly situation into a positive one you tend to look at things just a little bit differently. Everyone has a story to tell, but only few have testimonies.

The next day after being discharged from the hospital I wasn't feeling my best, but I thought that it would be a day that could finally help put my life back together again since I finally knew what was causing me pain and sickness. Oh, how I was mistaken.

Days and nights passed, and I just did not seem to be getting any better. In fact, I was getting worse by the day! We just couldn't figure out why since we thought that the problem had already been found. From the time I first started getting sick on Easter Sunday, until the time we found the blood clots from the MRI, I went from weighing two-hundred and fifty-five pounds to one hundred and seventy pounds and I was still losing weight. We could not begin to think what else could have been causing me to become so sick.

-

One day after waking up, I decided to remove my scarf so my hair could breathe. I got the shock of my life as I looked at my scarf and saw a handful of my hair. I immediately became worried and felt my hair. That's when the tears started to fall. I realized that my hair was falling out in chunks. I have always taken pride in my hair and it's something that I have always loved. So, the fact that I had just woken up to see my hair no longer attached to my scalp, was heartbreaking for me.

"Mom," I yelled at the top of my lungs trying to figure out in my head what the hell was going on and why my hair was sitting in my scarf and not on the top of my head. I waited a few seconds and yelled again, this time even louder. "Mommy!" I still received no answer. "Ma!!!" I received no answer from her yet again.

That's when I heard my dad yell, "Ti'Ocea what the hell wrong with you fool?"

Normally I would laugh at his crazy self, but this time I just couldn't seem to smile. "Dad, where is Mom? I need help," I yelled to him, hoping that someone would come up soon and help.

"Ti'Ocea what's wrong?" I heard my mom yell from downstairs.

"Ma, come here, I need help." I just wanted to figure out what was going on and fast. I heard my mother on the stairs coming up as fast as she could. As she came around the corner, I didn't even need to say anything because she saw exactly what I was calling her for. I was holding the chunks of hair in my hands with my head held down.

"OMG, what happened? And why is your hair in your hands?" she asked me with a look of disbelief and confusion on her face.

"I don't know, I just woke up and took off my scarf and all my hair was on my pillow and in my hands." I said all in one breath."

"Cam," she said calling for my dad to come and see what was going on.

"What y'all up here screaming for?" he asked as he turned the corner to see what all the fuss was about. "What the f***? What happened?" he asked as he looked between me and my mother trying to get the same questions answered as us.

"Looks like we are going to have to call Dr. Heather Lenior's office and get you an appointment scheduled immediately," my mother stated, as she headed to her room to get her phone and make the call to my primary care physician. Something else was going on and they were determined to figure it out no matter what. Someone was going to give them answers and fast. As I sat in the bed still in disbelief, I heard my father talking to me, but I could not process the words that were coming out of his mouth. I was lost in space.

"Ti'Ocea? Ti'Ocea? Hello, do you hear me? Are you ok?" I thought I was thinking those words, but later I found out it wasn't my thoughts, but my father's voice calling me. "Get up and get ready we are going to go see Dr. Heather Lenior today," my mother stated as they headed back to their room to get dressed. I could barely move as I was still stuck in my trance and trying so hard to come out of it, but it was hard. Finally, after five minutes, I was able to get up and get dressed but needed help because I was weak and unstable on my feet.

-

Slowly my parents led me downstairs to the car to take me to the doctor's office. As we made our way to Lac De Ville Blvd, all I could do is get lost in my thoughts that were overtaking me. I know I'm not supposed to question God, but God why is this happening to me? What else could be going wrong? Why me? Am I going to die? What is happening to me? I thought we had taken care of the problem. I should be getting better right now, not worse. Those were the thoughts that were going through my head during the car ride. I was so drowned in my thoughts that I didn't hear my mother calling for me to get out of the car. I jumped back into reality and opened the door to be helped out of the car and led up the stairs.

Immediately, when I opened the door the staff noticed that I was different and not myself. They noticed the drastic change in me since I had been coming there for a year and a half before this happened. I had gotten to know everyone quite well. "Mrs. Johnson come over and check her in and let her sit down in the chair," I heard the front desk staff say to my mother as I was being led to a chair.

It took about five minutes for my mother to check me in and take a seat to be waited to be called to the back. It took about another eight minutes for us to be called to the back. I got on the scale and realized I had dropped more than a few pounds since leaving the hospital, and that was not good. Nurse Melissa was the best and I always loved coming to see her because she was always the sweetest and cared about her patients. It's always good when you come to a doctor's office and all the staff treats you with respect and proves to you that they care for you no matter their position. It was such a blessing to be surrounded by so many wonderful people at a time like that.

"Ti'Ocea you don't look so good babe. What is going on with you?" Melissa asked me as she started typing something on her computer.

"Melissa how are you today?" my mother said. I knew she was getting ready to tell what was going on because this was what she did.

"I am good today, how are you?" Melissa replied. "What is going on with her? She does not look like she is getting any better than when we saw her last and this is worrisome," Melissa said and waited for a response from someone.

"Melissa, we took Ti'Ocea to the hospital and got to the bottom of the blood clots and got her on her medicine schedule along with seeing her hematologist. We thought that we had taken care of the problem, but it seems as if it is getting worse. Ti'Ocea is becoming very weak, she is unstable and today she woke up and all her hair was on her pillow and in her hands," my mother said as she looked at Melissa who was typing notes in her computer and trying to take everything in all at once.

"Oh, no this is not good. Let me get your blood pressure, so Dr. Heather Lenior can come in and talk with you all." Melissa stated, as she began taking my blood pressure and temperature. After she finished her routine, she told us that Dr. Heather Lenior would be in as soon as possible and that she was praying for me. With everything that was going on, prayer was the only thing that was getting us through. I remember when we were in the hospital and they had diagnosed me with the blood clots, I saw my mother break down like she has never broken down before. I told her, "Mom, it's going to be ok. I know it may not seem like it, but God is by our side. I am here for a reason. Turn the bible to Isaiah 54:17 and let's just read and sing the song."

The bible says in Isaiah 54:17: No weapon formed against me shall prosper, and every tongue that shall rise against thee in judgment thou shalt condemn. This is the heritage of the servants of the Lord, and their righteousness is of me, saith the Lord.

"No Weapon formed against me, shall prosper, it won't work. No Weapon formed against me shall prosper, it won't work. God will do what he said he will do, he's not a man that shall lie, he will come through!"

From there we just kept singing the song over and over and turning to that scripture everyday no matter how sick I was getting. Our faith was the only thing that was bringing our family through the hard times.

There was a knock then the door opened, and in came Dr. Heather Lenior with a concerned look on her face. She had always been a doctor who cared for me far better than any other doctor. She would make sure that she tried any and every possible solution there was to find answers for her patients. She was a blessing from God, and I was lucky to have a doctor such as her in my life.

"Ti'Ocea," Dr. Heather Lenior began, as she walked in the room with her computer in hand. She was always so thorough and made sure she never entered a room without her computer. "What is going on with you? You don't look so good since the last time I saw you," She stated. I didn't even open my mouth because I knew my mother was getting ready to tell her exactly what was going on with me, so I just sat back and listened.

She began to speak and repeat to her exactly what she had told to Melissa in the beginning. "Dr. Heather Lenior, well we took Ti'Ocea to the hospital after her MRI scan and thought we had gotten to the bottom of her being sick when they found the blood clots and put her on a routine medication schedule, along with seeing her hematologist. She continued. "We thought the problem had been taken care of, but it just seems to be getting worse. Ti'Ocea is becoming very weak, she is still losing weight tremendously, she is unstable on her feet and today she woke up and all her hair was on her pillow and in her hands. I am not sure why, but we would really like to figure out what is going on and get some true and accurate answers." She stated to Dr. Heather Lenior, as she was rapidly typing on her computer to make sure she documented everything.

"Let's check you out and see what is going on with you. I think that we are going to schedule an appointment with a rheumatologist, just to make sure there is not anything going on that is hereditary in your body, and to exhaust all possible options," she stated to us, as she began to do her routine exam on my body.

Dr. Heather Lenior ended up scheduling an emergency appointment with a rheumatologist by the name of Dr. Chad Gardenia. My appointment was set for the following day at ten in the morning. My dad and I were dressing up the next day to get ready for the appointment. One thing I can say is that I had the best family support anyone could ever ask for. If both could not be at the appointments, at least one was always there with me through it all, and for that I was and will forever be grateful.

At that moment in time, I didn't know what I would have done without them. We reached the rheumatologist office and I was a little anxious and nervous at the same time, because I had no idea what kind of problems they were going to find. But I was in God's hands, so no matter what they found I knew that I would be ok. I know sometimes we question what He does and why He does it, but God does everything for a reason, and it teaches us life lessons.

-

This had been our first time in a rheumatologist office and to be honest I didn't even know at first what rheumatology meant. I was just going with the flow. After reading and doing research, I found out that rheumatology is the study of your body and rheumatic diseases. Rheumatic diseases affect your bones, joints tendons, ligaments, and your muscles. It had me a little uneasy as I was reading the information because I was trying to figure out what was going inside of my body and why I was referred to see a rheumatologist.

So many thoughts run through your head daily, when you are facing different problems. It feels as if your brain never stops. For me, it just kept going and going until I would end up with headaches from asking myself these questions, questions that I may not ever find an answer to.

We went through the normal routine and questions as with any other doctor's appointment, but this time my dad was with me and was there to explain everything that transpired in my life.

A few minutes after the nurse had left, there was a knock on the door by who I was guessing was Dr. Chad Gardenia.

"Hello, come in," we said in unison, as a short, older, Chinese man walk through the door.

"Hello Ti'Ocea, I am Dr. Chad Gardenia. It is nice to meet you. I just wish it could have been under better circumstances," he said to me, as he reached out to shake our hands.

"Cameron," my dad said as they shook hands.

Dr. Chad Gardenia took a seat in his chair, ready to get started. "So, Dr. Heather Lenior told me a little bit about what was going on in the referral that she sent over, but I would like to hear from you guys. What has been going on with Ti'Ocea?"

"Well, Dr. Chad Gardenia," my dad began. It was so funny that anything that had to do with my health my mom and dad always spoke up before

I could even say anything, and my mom made sure she hit every detail even if it didn't matter. But, hey that's what parents are for and I didn't mind it one bit. "Ti'Ocea has been very sick since Easter Sunday and we have been back and forth to doctors and hospitals trying to figure out why she was getting so sick."

"Um hum," Dr. Chad Gardenia chimed in.

My father continued, "We thought we had found the problem when her PCP ordered an MRI and they found blood clots and pulmonary embolisms in her lungs that could have stemmed from the car accident she had with the 18-wheeler back in September of 2011. She was admitted into the hospital and they explained that she had blood clots and prescribed her Coumadin and Heparin to control her blood. We thought that was the heart of the problem, but it seems as if she is getting worse. She is in constant pain, she complains about her legs, she is very weak, she is unstable, and she woke up the other day with her hair falling out. So, you see this has been very challenging for us. We are just trying to find out what is going on with our daughter."

"I see. This must be very difficult for you all, especially you Ti'Ocea since you are the one enduring all this pain and to make matters worse, you are so young," Dr. Chad Gardenia stated to us. All I could do was shake my head and agree. "How about you come sit over here and let me do some tests to see if we can figure out what is causing your symptoms. Can you show me where on your legs it hurts?" Dr. Chad Gardenia asked me.

I pointed from my knee down to my ankle on both legs.

"And do they hurt every day?"

"Yes, they do. Sometimes it is like I can barely walk," I responded to him, hoping that he could find some answers and send us home with some information.

"Have you all ever heard of an auto immune disease?" Dr. Chad Gardenia asked both of us with me answering no and my dad answering yes. Neither one of us was very knowledgeable on the topic. "Well, an auto immune disease is a condition in which your immune system attacks your body," he started to explain. "Your immune system guards your body against germs like bacteria and viruses. But, when you have an auto immune disorder the immune system cannot tell the difference between good and bad cells, and release autoantibodies that end up attacking the good cells in your body. The symptoms of an auto immune disorder are, achy muscles, swelling, fevers, trouble concentrating, joint pain, extreme weight loss, hair loss, skin rashes etc. We think that you may have an auto immune disease called Sarcoidosis. Now normally, auto immune disorders are hereditary. Is there anyone in your family who suffered or suffers from an auto immune disorder?" Dr. Chad Gardenia asked us as we were still processing the information that was just given to us.

"No, not that we know of," I said, in a low weak tone.

"Well, what we are going to do is take some blood work from you and run it through the lab. Those results will give us a more definitive answer. From the signs that I am seeing and what you've shared with me, you have an auto immune disorder. So, I am going to put you on a medicine called

Plaquenil, also known as Hydroxychloroquine. It is used to treat most auto immune disorders. We want you to take that three times a day, until we figure out what you have and then we can go from there as to what are next steps are. Also, since you are so unsteady, I think it is best that you walk with a cane, until you can get better on your feet.

Just great! First, I have to deal with bruises and scars and now I must deal with walking with a cane. Ughhh…but whatever will help me get better, so be it. I knew nothing about an auto immune disease. Here I am healthy, maybe a little overweight in society's eyes, but I was healthy. I get hit by an eighteen-wheeler and my life just turns into what feels like hell within the blink of an eye. I mean what 23-year-old you know goes through this all within six months. I was so lost that I needed the Lord to guide me, but I just didn't know how. I was hurting, not just physically, but mentally and somewhat spiritually. I just didn't know what to do, but luckily, I was surrounded by spiritual people, so we were there to help uplift one another in tough times.

-

After we left doctor C's office, we went home and began to start the new medication plan to see if this would be of any help to me. We were glad that we had at least gotten somewhere, but it still was not set in stone and there were still more questions to be answered. My mother quit her job to take care of me since I needed hands on assistance and my father worked from home a lot more since I was getting worse. I dropped over one hundred pounds and was continually losing. I needed help bathing in the tub because I could barely move, and I had to now walk with a cane being that the auto immune disease took over my body and caused me to become very weak and unsteady. I felt as if I was suddenly a lot to deal with. How did this young, independent healthy girl go from working two to three jobs to not even being able to walk at all because of a car accident? It was so depressing to me.

Now, don't get me wrong, I am not saying that the car accident caused these problems. But what I am saying is that these problems were non-existent, until something traumatic happened and they took over my body.

A phone call pulled me out of my thoughts. "Hello, May I please speak with Ti'Ocea?" the lady on the other end of my phone said as I sat there trying to figure out who she was and why she was calling me.

"This is she. May I ask who is calling?" I asked with my phone now on speaker so that my parents could hear what was going on.

"Yes, this is Michelle from Dr. Chad Gardenia's office and I was calling to see if we could schedule another appointment with you so that Dr. Chad Gardenia can speak with you about the results from the blood work."

"Ok, yes ma'am what days do you have available, and what times?" I asked waiting for a response.

"Is there any way you will be able to come in tomorrow morning around ten o'clock?" She asked.

I looked to my parents to make sure that the time and day was ok before I confirmed the appointment. "Yes, ma'am, we will be there tomorrow at ten," I told her and ended the call.

Jeremiah 30:17 (NKJV)

"For I will restore health to you and heal you of your wounds, says the Lord..."

Chapter 4

The Diagnosis

It was nine o'clock in the morning and I was up struggling to get dressed for my appointment and probably annoying everyone else as I always do. Even though I know that they would never say that I was a lot, I knew that with what I had been going through it was a lot on them and I always felt a way about it. I was appreciative and was grateful for everything they endured during this rough time with me, and I prayed that I got better so that they could enjoy their lives without having to take care of me. I was ashamed at one point, but I knew that I had the best family support ever and it was something I cherished. Most people don't have family to be there when they are going through hard or rough times and they suffer alone. I was blessed to have mine right by my side every step of the way.

"Ti'Ocea, are you ready? We have to go!" I heard my dad yell from the bottom of the stairs making

his way up to help me down. I was ready to go
and receive whatever results they had, as long as
we figured out what was going on, I had accepted
it.

"Yes, Dad I am ready. Let's go." I said, as I made
my way to the stairs with my cane, ready to be led
down. It took us about five minutes to make it
downstairs and in the car, and about another
twenty minutes to make it to Dr. Chad Gardenia's
office.

It was a packed day in the office. There were people in there that looked to have been sitting there
for a while, judging by the looks on their faces. I
made my way to a chair, as my father checked us
in, and I laid my head back and closed my eyes.
Thoughts were running through my head non-
stop and I just could not get them turned off. I
tried everything but I think that I was so trauma-
tized from everything that had been going on, that
I just wanted answers to questions that no one
seemed to have.

Surprisingly, our wait wasn't long, and we were
ushered to a room. The nurse did her usual

routine of checking blood pressure, weight and listening to lungs, etc. Dr. Chad Gardenia was in the room within three minutes after the nurse left.

"Hi, Ti'Ocea and Cameron, it is nice seeing you again and as always I wish it was under different circumstances," Dr. Chad Gardenia stated, as he came in and shook our hands.

"So, I brought you in so that I could explain in person the results that we found with your blood work. It looks as if you have an auto immune disease called Sarcoidosis and Mixed Connective Tissue Disease. You also have what we call inflammatory arthritis. Sarcoidosis is an auto immune disease that affects multiple organs in your body, but mostly it affects your lungs and lymph glands. You may also have some inflamed tissue that can form in certain areas of your body. However, Mixed Connective Tissue Disease is characterized by some features that you may see in Systemic Lupus Erythematosus (SLE Lupus), Systemic Sclerosis, and Polymyositis. The symptoms that you have been experiencing such as your joint pain, swelling, muscle weakness, hair loss and numbness in fingers are only some of the symptoms found in patients with Mixed Connective Tissue Disease and Sarcoidosis. We did find that your Lupus levels were slightly elevated but not enough to diagnosis you with the disease," Dr. Chad Gardenia continued explaining everything, as we sat silently trying to grasp all the information being given to us.

"Now, the good thing is that the medication we are going to prescribe you treats mostly all of the auto immune diseases, so it should not have an effect on you if anything gets worse or changes," Dr. Chad Gardenia stated. Then he asked if there were any questions we had before he continued.

"Will this medication cause any other complications and how long will she have to take this medication?" My father asked.

"No, this medication should not cause any more complications. In fact, it should help decrease her pain and swelling that she has been experiencing. Now, because this is an auto immune disorder, she will have to be on this medication for the rest of her life and any other medication that is given to help treat her chronic illness. I am also going to prescribe her a muscle relaxer that will help decrease the joint pain that she has been experiencing. Now, there will be times where she will flare and no medication that she takes will help. Just let the flare happen and if it gets unbearable, go to the hospital."

"Dr. Chad Gardenia," I chimed in. "You stated earlier that the medication will help treat my chronic illness. Can you please explain to me what a chronic illness is? I am still trying to take all this information in and understand what everything means."

"Sure, I can explain. A chronic illness is basically just a long-term health condition that may not have a cure. It's a disease that persists for a long period of time. Now, I know this is difficult to process, especially since this is not hereditary for you, but I promise after you start your treatment process you will feel much better at least until a flare occurs. Yes, there will be complications and some days you'll feel extremely weak. But it is ok to call me or go to the hospital if you think something is not right. Please do not be afraid to call someone." Dr. Chad Gardenia mentioned as he stood up and typed something into his computer. "Ok, Ms. Hagins, I will see you back in about six months and hopefully you will be feeling better and I won't be seeing you with that cane anymore." Dr. Chad Gardenia said his goodbyes to us and moved on to his next patient.

The ride home was silent as we were both in our thoughts and trying to process all the information that was given to us. An auto immune disease? How could this be? It is not hereditary, so where did it come from? The rest of my life? I re-asked those questions repeatedly in my head trying to figure out how this could be, and why was this happening to me of all people.

That day after the doctor's appointment, we went home and explained what happened to the family. It was then that I decided I was not going to let this disease or anything else I had been through, stop me from reaching my dreams and accomplishing my goals. I was enrolled at Monroe Community College at the time that I got sick and I was determined to finish my degree one way or another. No matter what happened I was going to finish.

Surviving the Storms

That day I went to school and crawled into my classroom. Since there was no wheelchair around for me to use and I was experiencing excruciating pain, crawling was the only thing I could do. I crawled to the back of the class and leaned against the wall for support. My teacher Mrs. S noticed and told me to call who ever had dropped me off. At the time, I didn't ask why even though I was curious to know why she wanted to speak with my parent. I called my mom on the phone and told her to come inside of the classroom.

Mrs. S was one of my favorite teachers and she was always very understanding, especially when you are a student who did her work and made an effort to be in class. She had an awesome person-ality and she knew that life had a way of sneaking in and trying to break you, so certain circum-stances you couldn't control. My mother had just walked in the classroom as Mrs. S was waiting for class to begin and for some of the late arrivals to make it before the door shut. I guess today she was being extra generous. That door was normally shut at nine o'clock am on the dot. But, hey I wasn't complaining because I was always on time.

"Mrs. Hagins," Mrs. S called out to my mother.

"Johnson," my mother replied.

"Ok, I am sorry Mrs. Johnson. I am Mrs. S, Ti'Ocea's teacher and I wanted to speak with both of you privately, it will only be a few minutes." Mrs. S called for a wheelchair, so that I didn't have to crawl anywhere, and I could be comfortable. The wheelchair came to her room within seconds and I was helped into the chair and pushed outside of the door to join the conversation.

"What is going on with Ti'Ocea? I saw her crawling into the classroom." Mrs. S asked with a look of concern on her face.

"She has Sarcoidosis and Mixed Connective Tissue Disease, along with having a blood clotting disorder. She will be in a lot of pain for a while, but she is determined to finish her classes no matter what, even against my opinion," My mother said to Mrs. S as she looked to me and smiled gently.

"Listen, Ti'Ocea I know what it's like to live with pain and what Sarcoidosis can do to you. As I may not know physically, I know mentally what it can do as I have seen it tear my sister apart. Yes, she has Sarcoidosis and I know how that feels and what the pain looks like, just from being around her. I don't need you to be in class, to know what kind of grade I am going to give my students. You are a hard worker and dedicated. Please go home and take care of yourself and don't worry about class. I know what your grade is no matter if you are here or not. I know what kind of work you do and the time you put into it. Please go home and don't come back here until you have completely healed. You understand me, missy?" Mrs. S asked me as she got a tissue to wipe the tears from my eyes that had fallen during her speech.

"Thank you so much," my mother and I said in unison. We were speechless over what happened.

"No problem at all and I will see you at graduation soon fully back to yourself. Have a good day and please take it easy." Mrs. S stated to us, as she said goodbye and headed back to the classroom.

I was so grateful for her. She had really been a blessing to me. I was almost done with my classes and fell sick before I could finish. That day I went home and received emails from all my professors, telling me to take care of myself and that they were giving me an extension on the homework assignments, so I didn't have to worry about them for a while. Crawling into class that day showed that my determination is undeniable. I would and will do whatever it takes to achieve my dreams and goals. I have always been determined to achieve them by any means necessary.

Every day that I woke up was a struggle for me. I was depressed, but I never let it stop me. I was on double medication, taking shots in my stomach, going back and forth to doctor's appointments and my weight was constantly up and down. Oh, and to top it off I had to walk with my cane for six months before my body started to adjust back to normal and I could be stable enough to move without it.

One thing for sure and two things for certain, I had the upmost faith in the Lord. I had literally watched God bring me through one near death experience after another. The one thing that he never did was let me go. He had been my ultimate healer and if I was never sure about him before, I most definitely was certain about Him now. I've always been a believer of the most-high, but that belief becomes stronger when you experience something tragic. To some, He may not be real, but to others He is the only thing that stands between you and a casket.

Jeremiah 17:14 (NKJV)

"Heal me, O Lord, and I shall be healed;
save me, and I shall be saved, for You are my
praise."

Chapter 5

Living My Best Life

For the next seven months, after being diagnosed with Sarcoidosis, Mixed Connective Tissue Disease, and Inflammatory Arthritis, it took my faith in God to make it through. We never believe how much God is by our side until something tragic happens and He ends up saving us from being in a casket at an early age.

Walking with a cane was just as challenging as waking up every day getting shots in my stomach. I know, I know what everyone may be thinking. Getting shots in your stomach is not challenging. To some this may be true, but for those who don't do well with needles and are sensitive to pain, trust me when I tell you, it's challenging.

Every day I had to be extremely careful with everything I did and every move I made. Taking Coumadin, if I fell or hit anything on my body, I could have bled out internally. It was especially hard since I had to balance with a cane. To top it all off, I had to go get my blood drawn weekly to make sure my levels were stable. It was a "nightmare." By God's grace and mercy, I was alive and with my family, so I was not complaining. I did what I needed to do to get back on my feet.

Life felt normal again once I was able to go back to work at ADT Security Services and back to finishing my classes at Monroe Community College. I know there is no such thing as "normal," but when you are hanging on to the edge not knowing if you will live or die, when you have to learn how to do something over again that you were once able to do, anything outside what you are going through or have been through feels normal. Everyone will have different definitions of normal, but, normal is when you are in a routine that you have been in for the majority of your life.

"Ti'Ocea, on behalf of Monroe Community College, I am pleased to offer my congratulations upon the completion of your degree."

When I received that email after taking two months to submit my past due assignments, it was one of the proudest days of my life. In May of 2013, I graduated from Monroe Community College with my Associates of applied science degree in Criminal Justice. It was probably one of the best days of my life. I had finally, after so many challenges and complications interrupted my goals, graduated and finished what I set out to accomplish. But, stopping there wasn't in my agenda. I had already accomplished part of my dream, but I still had another to finish.

I enrolled in The State University of New York: College at Brockport. I was set to start in the fall of 2013. I was truly excited to be working towards my Bachelor's degree in Criminal Justice. Everything just seemed so unreal. I had gone from almost losing my life to finally graduating and achieving something I could be proud of in the years to come.

Life had been treating me well and to make things better I had recently received a job working for the State of New York: Finger Lakes Developmental Disabilities Service Office as a Direct

Support Assistant making $33,000 a year. I was itching to leave ADT and on May 30th, I would be heading over to the State of New York and would never look back.

1 Samuel 1:27 (NKJV)

"For this child I prayed, and the Lord has granted me my petition which I asked of Him."

Chapter 6

My Miracle

"Girl call him and don't be shy. Just be you,"
Crissy said as she had just given me the number to the cousin of the guy she was dating. I guess he was looking for someone to chill with and asked if she had any friends. Of course, she chose me, and at first, I was upset with her just to be giving me up like that and not even telling me nothing about it. What I didn't know was that he would turn out to be my happily ever after.

Ring, Ring! Ring, Ring!

"Hello," a deep voice answered on the other end of the phone.

"Hello, may I speak with D?" I asked not knowing what I was about to get myself into.

"This D, who dis?"

"This is TiOcea, Crissy's friend she told you about." I said with a little bit of nerves in my stomach. Why, I didn't know, but I always tend to get like that when I speak to men. Just something that has always happened with me.

"Oh yeah, what's up shorty?" he said to me in a deep but soft voice and that was the start of a long conversation, a five-and-a-half-year relationship and one child. We talked night and day, day and night. Hours on top of hours. Days turned into weeks, weeks turned into months and months turned into years. Our chemistry and attraction was like no other and it allowed us to create a sustainable and stable relationship. We not only became lovers; we became best friends. If you saw one of us, you saw the other. It was like Bonnie and Clyde. Then something happened that changed our lives forever.

-

"Ma'am, Ma'am? Are you ok?" Asked the EMT worker who was outside of my car door trying to get me out of the smashed car. Anyone who has ever lived anywhere up north, knows that when it snows and ices, it is no joke and you must be extremely careful when driving. I was on my way to work driving slowly as the snow was falling hard making the visibility of the roads extremely difficult to see. Boom! That was the sound of my car hitting the guard rail after hitting a patch of ice and spinning out of control.

Boom! That was my car hitting the same guard rail again after doing another 360-spin hitting another patch of ice. Boom! That was my car hitting the guard rail a third and final time. Other drivers stopped to help and make sure I was ok, while one called the police and ambulance. Thank God they did not take that long to get there, because I was in pain and ready to get out that car.

Woo-woo-woo! Those were the sounds of the sirens I heard coming down the street to my rescue. In my mirror, I saw the ambulance slide on a patch of ice as they tried to pull over to come and help me. Behind them was the police and fire truck. I was so grateful to have saw them.

"Ma'am, Ma'am are you ok?" The EMT worker asked as they opened my car door to help me on to the stretcher. Luckily, I was not hurt as bad because the passenger side of my car got the most damage, but I was still in pain and had to go to the hospital.

While I was waiting for medical help, I called my parents to let them know I had been in an accident and they had arrived just shortly after medical help came on scene. We arrived at the Hospital and I was immediately taken to a room. My mom, father and uncle had already made it to the hospital before we arrived. I was so luckily to have such wonderful family support.

"Ms. Hagins, my name is Tina. I am going to be your nurse today. I'm going to go ahead and give you an IV. Can you please verify your information for me?" Tina asked as I moved to make myself comfortable with that awful neck brace on. I could not wait until it was taken off, I hated it with a passion, but I knew it was precaution and needed to be done.

"Ms. Hagins, what happened?" Tina asked me as I began telling her what had just taken place. "Well, I'm glad you are ok! Let's go ahead and give you an IV to start some fluids for you. Then, we must collect a urine sample just to make sure all is ok. Once that is completed, we can see about getting you an x-ray so that we can get your neck brace removed and give you some meds."

"Ok, that sounds good to me," I stated as I watched my dad walk in the room.

My uncle, mom and dad had followed us to the hospital, as soon as we had left the accident scene. My uncle and mom were outside of the room, but my dad had just come in the room. As soon as I was about to say something to him the nurse walked in the room, with this look on her face that had me worried like something had happened.

"Ms. Hagins, I have some news for you," I heard her say as I saw my dad walking towards the door with his finger up and him saying, "I know what this is. Let me go get ya' mama!"

"Ms. Hagins, congratulations you're pregnant!" She said to me.

I just stared at her for a long minute trying to take in the words that she just said to me. This couldn't be. The doctors told me I could never have kids.

How can this be? No, No, they told me I could never have kids. This must be a joke. These thoughts were consuming me until I heard my mom come in and interrupt my train of thought.

"What's going on T?" she said as I looked at her not prepared to tell her the very words that was just spoken to me. Why? I still don't know. I was 24 and I had my own job, home, etc.… but I still didn't know why I was scared to say the words.

"I'm pregnant mom! She just told me that they tested my urine and it came back positive."

"Well, ma'am test it again!" she said and although I was in tears, all I could do was laugh, because I had just said the same thing to the nurse right before my mother walked in the room. We thought alike. I told that lady that she had mixed up my urine and needed to retest it again and fast. (Laughing out loud.)

I still was not convinced that I was pregnant because I had been told that I could never have kids, so I just couldn't believe that I had received a positive pregnancy test.

"Ms. Hagins, we have retested the urine three times and it is coming back positive for pregnancy." The nurse said to me as I was still laying on the bed crying and laughing. My uncle had come into the room and joined me and my mother as I sat there just apologizing. For what? I didn't know. "I am so sorry Mom. I am sorry!" I don't know why I was saying I was sorry. I guess I was happy and sad at the same time, because I was always trying to do everything the right way and wanted to make sure I made my parents proud. I worried that having a baby would disappoint them. But I was mistaken!

"Ti'Ocea, it's ok it happens. You are a grown woman!" My mother said to me as she sat there looking at me.

"It's ok baby!" My uncle said to me. I was in such a big shock, that I was just trying to take it all in. I was told by the nurse that I had to go into an x-ray. I was waiting for transport to come and take me back, when I decided to call the father of our, soon to be child, and tell him the news that I had just received. He answered on the first ring and I was relieved to hear his voice. His voice always soothed me, especially when I am upset or just need someone to talk to.

"Hello, what's up babe?" he said to me as I silently prepared myself to tell him the news.

"Babe, are you sitting down? Because I have something to tell you?"

"Girl just say what you have to say!" he said to me and all I could do was chuckle, because I knew that always made him mad. He is a get to the point and don't waste no time kind of man.

"Babe, I am pregnant!" I blurted out and expecting to get an overjoyed reaction, all I got was, "Oh word!"

Thought back on a conversation we'd previously had… "I have always wanted children. It was something that I said I wanted, a family. I tried so many times to have children. But every relationship I was in and my woman got pregnant, she ended up having a miscarriage. The one time I had the chance to be a father, I was robbed of that chance. My ex-girlfriend had an abortion, taking away the one thing that I wanted so badly, and there was nothing that I could do about it."

-

Those were the words that he said to me in the beginning of our relationship. So, his reaction was consistent to what he had previously gone through. He did not want to get his hopes up, until he knew that this baby was going to make it to full term. He was skeptical and I understood it, especially since I would be a high-risk pregnancy due to my previous health problems.

That day was the start of something special for us. Man had told us that we could not have any kids and we were torn. That was disheartening to us. We met one another and God had a different plan. Our miracle baby was happening.

-

"Ok, Ti'Ocea I need you to push and hold down because he is coming." I heard my OB doctor say, as I sat on that bed trying as hard as I could to push this baby out of me. I wanted him out, but the pain was just too much and I was getting tired of pushing. It was all too much.

"Push, Ti'Ocea, push!" she said again.

"I can't no more. I'm tired. Just push him back in! I feel like I'm about to poop!" I screamed at her because I couldn't take the pain or the feeling. An epidural was out of the question for me since I had a previous blood clotting disorder, so I had to give birth to my son naturally.

"One more big push!" I heard Dr. S say as I pushed down as hard as I could and heard my baby cry for the first time. Tears came to my eyes. After carrying him for forty weeks, I finally heard him cry, and it was the best moment of our lives.

God allowed me to deliver a healthy five-pound, nine-ounce baby boy who was born on August 7, 2014 7:15pm.

Sometimes we put so much faith in man, that we count out what God can do. Man had told me one thing, but God had done another after having relations with a few ex-boyfriends and never getting pregnant. I had believed what man said. But we must not count out God, and how He is the ultimate decider in our fate.

It's not over, until God

says it over...

Chapter 7
C. Difficile Colitis

Web MD and medicinenet.com defines C. difficile colitis, often called c difficile or c diff, as a bacterium that can cause symptoms ranging from diarrhea to life threating inflammation of the colon. C. difficile causes colitis by producing toxins that damage the lining of the colon. The symptoms of c. difficile colitis are fever, diarrhea, dehydration, and abdominal pain. Each year in the united states of America, about a half of million people get sick from c. difficile colitis. C diff infections have become more frequent.

"Beep, Beep, Beep." Those were the sounds of the machines that was keeping my lifeless body alive.

I came into the hospital to be treated for the flu and ended up with machines working to keep me alive. I had been to multiple doctor's appointments, but nothing seemed to be working.

But wait! Before I get to that part let me tell you how I got here and how we found out about c-difficile colitis.

It was Thursday morning and my parents were getting ready to go on a trip to find a home for us in Charlotte, NC. That morning I woke up and was getting out of the bed to get myself together for the morning. I stood up and was on my way to the bathroom when I had a huge bowl movement in the middle of the hallway floor. It had happened so fast that no one was prepared for it. But, how can someone be prepared for anything like this anyway? I was so sick that anything could happen.

My dad and child's father rushed to get some paper towels and cleaning supplies, while my sister helped me into the bathroom. It was the scariest thing that I had seen. My parents left to go on their trip but were skeptical of leaving me since everything started to happen little by little. Later that night I was taken into the hospital because I was getting worse and it was time for some answers. My parents were not accepting just anything, they wanted to know what was wrong with their daughter.

The emergency room was packed that night as it always is, and the people were flocking in and out. Some looking defeated and others looking aggravated due to the long wait with all the people that were in the waiting area. This was going to be a long night and I had to prepare myself for it.

"Ms. Hagins," I heard my name called for registration, but because I was so sick, my baby's father wheeled me up to the front and helped me check in. We sat in the waiting room for about 45 minutes before we were called to the back.

"Ms. Hagins, can you tell me your full name and birthdate please?" The nurse in the pretty pink scrubs said to me, as she led us back to the room to get my vitals.

The attending physicians that night decided that admitting me to the hospital was in my best interest and the way I was feeling and fading my family was not going to accept anything less. Something was going to be done and soon.

Never would I have thought in a million years that I would once again be faced head to head with death.

"Why are you doing that?" I heard my dad say faintly as I watched the nurse take my vitals lying down, sitting up and eventually standing.

"They normally do this when they are in the process of discharging patients," Nurse Becca stated as I fell back on to the bed having fainted when I stood up.

"Well, Mrs. Becca, I don't care who you have to get whether it's the doctor, social worker, or whoever, but my daughter is not leaving this hospital until we have a care plan or a diagnosis." My dad said to her with an authoritative, but caring voice.

As we sat in the room waiting for someone to walk through the doors with some answers of what could be causing me to become so sick, I just sat and thought about it. My throat was so sore and closed up to the point where I could not speak, my eyes felt swollen shut and my nose felt as if someone had taken something and hit it until it closed. What was causing me to become this ill? How did this happen? What is going to happen from here? Am I going to die? How can I protect my son if I am dead? There were so many thoughts going through my head and the questions began to scare me because I was not getting any better. If anything, I was fading away little by little and at this point, all I had to lean on was my father above!

Knock, Knock!

The knock on the door interrupted my thoughts. "Come in."

Dr. Wong entered the room. "Ms. Hagins, Mr. Johnson, I am Dr. Wong. I'm sorry that we have to meet under these unfortunate circumstances. My staff tells me that you have some concerns about your health."

That started the beginning of this roller coaster ride, called health. From that day on, I just kept fading. Test after test, blood draw after blood draw doctors and nurses kept trying but kept coming up short. Nothing. Until one doctor told my parents, "I promise that I am going to get to the bottom of this. I promise she is going to be ok." That doctor hit the nail on the head and ending up changing our lives forever.

John 10:10 (NKJV)

"The thief does not come except to steal, and to kill, and to destroy. I have come that they may have life, and that they may have it more abundantly."

Chapter 8

Surviving the Storm

"Promise me that you will come back to me."

Those words pierced through me as I was fading away in the night. Doctors had finally come through and found a diagnosis. Something called C. Difficle Colitis. I don't know where the hell this came from, but I knew this was nothing but the devil and all he was trying to do was take me out.

"Ms. Hagins, it's time!" The doctors were prepping me for surgery and getting ready to put me to sleep for a good night's rest. They gave me some time to say goodbye to my family and it was the hardest thing that I could do. Instead of crying, I was trying to comfort my family members who were standing over me in tears.

"It's going to be ok. I'm going to be alright!" I said faintly to everyone.

The only one who was missing was my mother. She was out with my son trying to take care of him. He ended up getting sick and she had to stay with him in the hospital.

"Tanya, hurry up! They are taking her back. Get here now!" I heard my dad say to her as he was trying to make sure she had a chance to see me before I went back for a surgery that could possibly save my life or put me in the grave. The doctors had told my family that my organs were shutting down on me and the C Diff had perforated my colon. I had a twenty percent chance at surviving with or without the surgery. No one wants to hear that their baby may not make it. Those words left my family afraid of losing me.

"Mrs. Johnson, you have 30 seconds to talk. We have to take her, and we have to take her now." The doctors had given me my medicine and I was going to be out in just a few seconds.

"Baby promise me you will come back to me. Promise me you will come back to me," my mother said crying as she only had a few seconds to talk because it was time to make or break my life.

"I promise Mom. I'm coming back." And just like that I faded away in the dark never to return.

Well... so I thought!

-

Someone help me! Someone help me! Please! I am being taken. Mommy... Daddy help! Those are the thoughts that were going through my head as I was rolling on something that seemed like a cart going somewhere unfamiliar. My eyes began to flutter, and I began to see things quickly. I must have been medicated, but just not enough because I was beginning to awaken. Something was wrong, and I was determined to figure it out. I tried to move my arms and legs and realized I was being held down. Help me, someone please help! I tried to scream, but something was stuck in my throat and I couldn't scream for help.

Now I am worried. Someone had me and I needed to get out of there fast. I started to move my legs and arms to break free from my grip, but the restraints were too tight and too strong. Someone help me! I tried screaming again and opened my eyes to see where I was, but just as I was trying to get them fully open, I was hit with this thing called sleep and my fight to get free had just killed me.

-

Family had flown in from all over and gathered in the waiting area of the hospital. My family would not leave the waiting room until they knew that I was ok. No one would even speak words, because at the time there were none to be spoken. Doctor Jones had come into the waiting room many times to pray with my family and to make sure that they were ok. He was one of the good ones. Before he left for the day, he had told my parents,

"She's going to be ok." She is in the Lords hands and I can feel it. Relax with ease and call me if you need me."

That was the last time they had saw or talked to him. We think that the hospital may have transferred him.

-

I had awakened from what I thought was a dream and immediately ended up realizing it was reality. So much had changed just within a few hours. I had felt like my body had left me and I was just here on this earth like a zombie, not feeling anything.

My depression was at an all-time high. I thought I was done. Ready to leave never to return, but God had another plan. It was crazy because I had gone from being a somewhat normal human being to being laid up in ICU on life support not knowing if I was going to live or die. No matter whether I made it through or not, my life would never be the same again. The traumatic and horrific experience was something that I wouldn't wish on my worst enemies.

After pulling through with what they thought would be my last few hours on life support, depression had hit me worse than anyone could ever imagine. I thought I was ready to leave this Earth never to return, but God had another plan.

It was crazy because just a month ago, I was working and living the good life and then a month later

I'm in ICU fighting to stay alive. The next words from the doctors to my parents could have been enough to make anyone upset and lose whatever little hope they were holding on to.

"Mr. and Mrs. Johnson," doctors called out and didn't wait for a response, they kept talking. "We are glad that your daughter made it through the surgery successfully, but because her organs are still not working, these next twenty-four hours are going to be crucial. If she does not make any progress, then you will have to pull the plug on her and say good-bye."

Goodbye was not in anyone's vocabulary! My doctors had counted me out, but my father above is the God of healing and ultimately it is His decision on whether I stayed alive on this Earth or join Him in the heaven's above.

Isaiah 41:10: "So do not fear, for I am with you; do not be dismayed, for I am your God. I will strengthen you and help you; I will uphold you with my righteous right hand." (NIV)

This disease had cost me a lot. Yes, as I was more than grateful to be alive, but it took me a long time to get back to the "I'm Alive, so that's all that matters" mindset. I had to work hard to get to that point. What do I mean by work hard? It does not mean physically working at a job, it means that with all the challenges that I endured, I had to fight my way past my challenges. I had to overcome my obstacles and fight my way back to my life. My family. My Son.

Bruises filled my body and keloids covered my legs. An ileostomy bag hung over the side of my stomach. Black marks covered every inch of my body from head to toe due to my skin popping from being pumped with so much blood and fluids. My head was the size of a watermelon and my legs were as big as two turkeys put together. My body had swollen ten times the size of the normal.

Silence filled the room. Doctors and nurses coming in and out to check on me asking questions, but no words could leave my lips. T.V. playing, but no words can be heard. My family had to push doctors to get me out of the bed and the funk that I was in. Thoughts clouded my mind that were not of God, but at the time I didn't want to live. I was ready to take my life, so I thought, so talking to people and being happy was something that at the time was the furthest from my mind.

Deuteronomy 31:8: "The Lord himself goes before you and will be with you; he will never leave you or forsake you. Do be afraid; do not be discouraged." (NIV)

After spending over a month in the hospital, after being counted out by my own doctors, after my depression kicked in and the enemy played with my thoughts and feelings, it was time for me to finally start my recovery process. It was time for me to take my life back one day at a time. If I didn't fight for myself, no one else would fight for me. I had to push and fight my way back to my life and my family.

Was it going to be easy? No! In fact, it was more than just difficult. From the physical therapy and learning how to walk again, to my nursing staff and my sister putting me in the shower to rip off the bandages from my body that was left on me by the hospital and having to listen to my mom cry in the other room, because she could hear the screams from me through the wall. Nothing was easy! The recovery process was something beyond difficult. There were times my depression kicked backed in and I wanted to give up. I didn't want to keep going through the process, but then I remembered that taking my life was not what God wanted. He would have done it Himself when I was sick and fighting to stay alive, if that's where He wanted me to be. He saved my life for a reason.

So, from that moment forward, I fought, and I fought hard. I looked at my son and I knew that if I didn't fight for anything else, that I would fight for him. He would be my reason I stay here on this Earth. He would be the motivation for me to keep pushing.

Sometimes we fight the wrong battles. We fight things that are either out of our control or can't be fought, but the things that we can fight, we make excuses about why we can't fight them. I'm glad that I fought. I'm glad I reached into my inner faith and leaned on the one man who I knew would help me get through this. And He did! He helped me conquer and overcome my obstacles. He helped me survive my storms and bring me back to myself one day at a time.

Because of God's help, Ti'Ocea is back and here to stay!

Chapter 9

A Letter to you

Dear Reader,

So, you may be asking yourself why would I write this story? And why would I tell you about me when no one even knows who I am? I write this story because it's my truth. Because there is someone out there who needs to hear this story. There is that one person who needs someone like myself, to tell their story, so that they can be ok. It's hard to talk to someone who does not understand what you have gone through... the pain that you have experienced firsthand.

Yes, some may have been there with you through it all, but still no one knows your pain. No one understands how much your faith has been tested because you feel as if there is no other reason to live on this Earth since this traumatic experience, but it is.

Take me for example, through all my obstacles, trials and tribulations, I thought that leaving this Earth was the best thing for me, but I was sadly mistaken. My family and friends have been my rock. I don't what I would have done without them. When you have a great support system, everything seems to be much better and it becomes so much easier.

My family came in from all over to stay by myside while I fought through my battles. Some from North Carolina, California and everyone else right from our hometown. They prayed by my bed side day in and day out. They filled the hospital waiting area with pillows and blankets and never left until I was in the clear. They wrote letters, cards, filled my room with balloons and cried tears with me , all while nursing me back to health and staying positive through it all.

Yet, even through all the things that they have done for me and all the support they have given, they don't and will never understand that trauma that I experienced. Truth be told, no one will ever understand unless they have been through it. But even people who have gone through challenges similar to yours, will never understand the pain, obstacles, trials or tribulations you overcame, because no two people are alike. No two people have the same situations. And that is okay because that is how God made us. He knows everyone will not be able to handle your situation, just as you will not be able to handle theirs.

We all have testimonies and stories to tell, but if we are not here to fight and live them, they will just be another memory. They will not matter, and you will just be another person who survived a storm, but no one will ever know why or how. No matter how many people surrounded me in the ICU or how many were involved with nursing me back to health, ultimately the decision to live and fight was mine and mine alone, just like your decision is yours.

Stay tuned for more about my life these days and I might bring along some people to tell their story.

About the Author

Ti'Ocea Hagins is a native of Rochester, N.Y. where she lived all her life with her mother, father, and younger brother and sister. She also has an older step-brother that resides in California. Ti'Ocea is a high school graduate of Nazareth Academy High School in Rochester, NY. Ti'Ocea became ill in her early adult life, when she was told that she would not be able to have children. On August 7, 2014, she was blessed with her now, 5-year-old son Jhaceon.

Despite her illnesses, she successfully obtained her Associate's degree in Criminal Justice from Monroe Community College. She then went on to complete her Bachelor's degree in Criminal Justice and Foren-sic Science from Brockport State College in Brock-port, NY. Currently, Ti'Ocea is battling an autoim-mune disease called Lupus and despite her disability she continues to be dedicated to any and everything she does. Her most recent accomplishment is her in-duction into the first-ever Greek Lettered diseased based organization. A sorority for women with Lu-pus, Lambda Sigma Sigma Lupus Sorority, Inc. Through her faith, she remains to be very active and committed to living a normal life. Currently, she re-sides in North Carolina with her family.